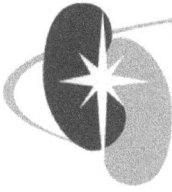

Renal Diet HQ IQ
Teaching You To Master Your Health

Anemia and Chronic Kidney Disease: Signs, Symptoms, and Treatment for Anemia in Kidney Failure

Book 11

By Mathea Ford, RD/LD

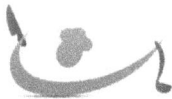

RENALDIET
HEADQUARTERS
BY HEALTHY DIET MENUS FOR YOU

Purpose and Introduction

What I have found through the emails and requests of my readers is that it is difficult to find information about a pre-dialysis kidney lifestyle that is actionable. I want you to know that is what I intend to provide in all my books.

I wrote this book with you in mind: the person with kidney problems who does not know where to start or can't seem to get the answers that you need from other sources. This book will provide information that is applicable to a predialysis kidney disease lifestyle.

Who am I? I am a registered dietitian in the USA who has been working with kidney patients for my entire 15 + years of experience. Find all my books on Amazon on my author page: http://www.amazon.com/Mathea-Ford/e/B008E1E7IS/

My goals are simple – to give some answers and to create an understanding of what is typical. In this series of 12 books, I will take you through the different parts of being a person with pre-dialysis kidney disease. It will not necessarily be what happens in your case, as everyone is an individual. I may simplify things in an effort to write them so that I feel you can learn the most from the information. This may mean that I don't say the exact things that your doctor would say. If you don't understand, please ask your doctor.

I want you to know, I am not a medical doctor and I am not aware of your particular condition. Information in this book is current as of publication, but may or may not have changed. This book is not meant to substitute for medical treatment for you, your friends, your caregivers, or your family members. You should not base treatment decisions solely on what is contained in this book. Develop your treatment plan with your doctors, nurses and the other medical professionals on your team. I recommend that you double-check any information with your medical team to verify if it applies to you.

In other words, I am not responsible for your medical care. I am providing this book for information and entertainment purposes, not medical diagnoses. Please consult with your doctor about any questions that you have about your particular case.

Table of Contents

Introduction

Anemia is one of the most common symptoms of chronic kidney disease (CKD). In fact, more than half of the individuals with end-stage renal disease suffer from anemia. Anemia occurs when the body is unable to produce enough red blood cells. In CKD, the diseased kidneys find it difficult to create enough erythropoietin (EPO), a hormone that is necessary for the creation of the red blood cells.

In CKD, it is possible for anemia to occur even before the kidneys fail, although it's more common for those in the advanced stages. It is also extremely common for individuals on dialysis to suffer from anemia.

Although it's often considered a symptom of CKD, anemia is serious in its own right and steps should be taken to correct and manage it. Many people with anemia suffer from a decreased quality of life, especially since common symptoms include fatigue, dizziness, decreased energy levels, and insomnia. If left untreated, anemia can even cause heart problems and increase the risk for heart disease and stroke.

Luckily, there are several blood tests that can be performed to evaluate and find the cause of the anemia. Once the cause has been established, treatment can commence. Treatment can consist of oral iron supplements, EPO therapy, and certain dietary changes. The good news is that anemia treatment is considered very effective and most patients experience a decrease of symptoms and an improved quality of life once they start treatment.

In the following book, we'll go over the causes of anemia, the common symptoms, lab tests that are used to diagnose and evaluate the anemia, and common treatment options that are used to manage it in the patient with chronic kidney disease.

What is anemia?

Anemia basically occurs when the body is unable to make adequate amounts of red blood cells. The red blood cells are important since they transport oxygen to the rest of the body, especially the vital organs. The oxygen that is transported by the red blood cells performs many functions, such as changing the glucose that is derived from the food we consume into the energy our body needs and uses. When there aren't a lot of red blood cells available, there isn't a good supply of oxygen on hand to perform these functions. As a result, the vital organs and the body's tissues can't do their jobs. This is a big problem for organs such as the heart and kidneys.

Anemia is a common problem in individuals who have chronic kidney disease, mostly due to the low amounts of the hormone erythropoietin in the body or an iron deficiency. When the body is experiencing low oxygen levels, a signal is sent to the kidneys to release erythropoietin (EPO). The hormone itself is necessary because it signals the bone marrow to produce more red blood cells (RBCs). When the body has the right amount of red blood cells then the oxygen can be transported. Unhealthy kidneys, however, might not make any EPO at all (or make very little) and this is a problem because the next step in the cycle does not occur.

The chain of events might look something like this:

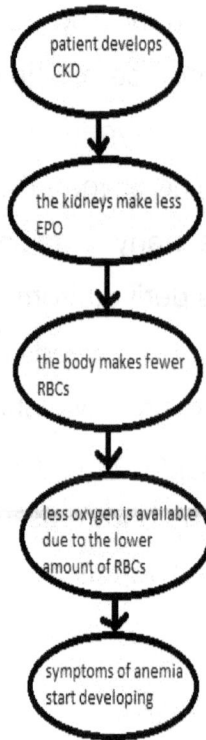

```
         ┌──────────────────┐
         │  patient develops │
         │       CKD         │
         └──────────────────┘
                  │
                  ▼
         ┌──────────────────┐
         │ the kidneys make  │
         │    less EPO       │
         └──────────────────┘
                  │
                  ▼
         ┌──────────────────┐
         │ the body makes    │
         │   fewer RBCs      │
         └──────────────────┘
                  │
                  ▼
         ┌──────────────────┐
         │ less oxygen is    │
         │ available due to  │
         │ the lower amount  │
         │     of RBCs       │
         └──────────────────┘
                  │
                  ▼
         ┌──────────────────┐
         │ symptoms of       │
         │ anemia start      │
         │  developing       │
         └──────────────────┘
```

Iron levels

Healthy iron levels are critical in order for the body to function properly. In order to create healthy red blood cells, the body needs iron. A lot of the iron is in hemoglobin, a protein that transports the oxygen in the blood. Anemia can be characterized by low levels of hemoglobin, that leads to low levels of iron. Both can lead to anemia, just like decreased erythropoietin levels.

When treating anemia, it's necessary to know the body's iron levels. Some of the common blood tests that are carried out include: hematocrit (Hct), hemoglobin (Hgb), serum ferritin, total iron-binding capacity (TIBC), serum iron, and transferrin saturation (TSAT). These test results can help the doctor establish the cause of an iron deficiency.

Serum Ferritin. Ferritin is a protein that sticks to iron and assists the body in the storage of iron. The body usually stores a certain amount of iron since it's so important for the body to function. Normal values are around 12 - 300 ng/mL (nanograms per milliliter of blood) for men and 12 - 150 ng/mL for women. For individuals who are on dialysis, the target range is 100-1,200 ng/mL. If the levels are low it could mean that the body doesn't have enough iron reserves. Still, while low levels are usually an indication of iron-deficiency anemia, high levels are not ideal either. If levels are too high it could indicate hemolytic anemia. Hemolytic anemia occurs when blood cells are damaged and bone marrow can't replace red blood cells that are being damaged. This can occur during dialysis.

It's important for ferritin levels to be within the proper range. If there is too much in the body then it can cause damage to the vital organs as well.

Total Iron Binding Capacity. The total iron binding capacity (TIBC) measures the level of transferrin, a protein that carries iron, in the blood. A TIBC measures how much transferrin in the body is transporting the iron, or if it is carrying it at all. A high TIBC is usually an indication of iron-deficiency anemia while a low level might reflect anemia caused by a chronic disease. In iron-deficiency anemia, the TIBC is high since iron stores are low. In anemia where chronic diseases are concerned, the TIBC is frequently below normal due to the fact that the iron stores are elevated. It's an inverse relationship because inflammation and certain chronic diseases can make it difficult for the body to be able to use the iron that is being stored. It's not just a matter of the body lacking the iron, it's a problem of the body knowing what to do with the iron that it has on hand.

Reticulocyte Count. Reticulocytes are young red blood cells, and the Reticulocyte count shows the rate of red blood cell creation. Normally, the upper limit is about 100,000/mL. If bleeding is not determined to be a cause then a low count might indicate production problems within the bone marrow. If there is a very high count then it could mean that red blood cells are being destroyed which could reflect a different type of anemia.

Serum Iron. The serum iron measures the quantity of iron that is in the blood. An average serum iron is 60 - 170 mcg/dL (micrograms per deciliter). Anything lower could mean the body has developed iron-deficiency anemia. High levels could indicate vitamin B12 or B6 deficiency, hemolytic anemia, hemolysis (your body doesn't have enough healthy red blood cells), or that your body is retaining too much iron.

Vitamin Deficiencies. The doctor may also order tests to check for vitamin B12 and folate deficiencies. The Schilling test is used to decide if the body is properly absorbing vitamin B12. Vitamin B12 is important since your body needs it in order to make red blood cells. Red blood cells, of course, carry oxygen through the body. Likewise, folate is also necessary for the generation of new red blood cells and without adequate supply of folate (also known as folic acid) the body simply isn't able to make the amount of red blood cells it needs.

The values of these various tests can vary depending on the lab. Most labs have their own range that is considered "normal" but they will still supply the results to the doctor in order for him or her to make the best possible decision regarding the anemia evaluation.

What Causes Anemia?

There are several reasons why an individual with CKD might suffer from anemia, but diet is often one of the first underlying causes that a doctor might investigate. Because individuals in the early stages of CKD are advised to limit the protein they consume, they might not get enough iron and B vitamins from their diets which could lead to anemia.

Iron deficiency is frequently seen in those CKD, especially those on dialysis, because of considerable loss of blood due to recurrent blood tests and blood that stays in the dialysis tubing. Anemia can also occur in CKD since the kidneys are not able to filter the waste like they should, and the waste stays in the bloodstream, decreasing the lifespan of the red blood cells and causing anemia as well.

Additional reasons why patients with CKD might suffer from anemia include:

- **EPO deficiency**: Healthy kidneys produce erythropoietin (EPO) a hormone that causes the bone marrow to produce the right amount of red blood cells that are necessary to transport oxygen to the rest of the body. In CKD, though, the kidneys usually don't produce enough EPO so the bone marrow doesn't produce as many red blood cells.

- **Other vitamin deficiencies**: Folic acid and vitamin B12 deficiencies are often tested for in patients to ensure they are getting the correct diagnosis. Megaloblastic anemia is characterized by a lot of big, young, and dysfunctional red blood cells. Megoblastic anemia is often caused by a vitamin B12 deficiency, which is a common occurrence in chronic kidney disease.

- **Blood loss**: Some patients, especially those who undergo transplants and other surgeries, might suffer from anemia due to blood loss. Those on dialysis often suffer from anemia for the same reason.

- **Bone marrow suppression**: Since the tranferrin levels in patients with CKD are less than they should be, it is often difficult for the body to transfer the iron that is taken in by the body to the bone marrow.

- **Iron not released**: Macrophages are important because they are cells that form to help the body fight off infections and inflammation. They take iron from the red blood cells and use the iron in the body in a healthy individual. However, for those with CKD, the disease can block the iron from being released so that the macrophages are unable to scavenge it.

Decreased Erythropoietin Production

If an individual has lost at least half of their normal kidney function and has a low hematocrit (the proportion of their red blood cells to the complete amount of their blood), their anemia is probably caused by a decreased erythropoietin (EPO) production. According to the guidelines, if there isn't a cause of anemia detected in CKD patients, and the serum creatinine is 2.0 mg/dL, then the anemia is almost certainly caused by an EPO deficiency. The possibility of anemia associated with EPO deficiency increases once the kidney function starts to decline since the kidneys are no longer able to create adequate quantities of EPO. Of course, it is still possible for anemia to develop fairly early in CKD, too.

People who have diabetes are at a higher risk of developing anemia at an earlier stage since they're more likely to have low levels of erythropoietin. In comparison to those who have a similar GFR (the glomerular filtration rate) and erythropoietin level, those who also suffer from type 2 diabetes are normally more anemic, according to the Nice Clinical Guidelines (Anaemia management in people with chronic kidney disease (CG114) 2011).

When Does Anemia Occur?

Those on dialysis

Individuals who are on dialysis often face anemia because they need extra iron in their bodies. This is because they either lack foods that are rich in iron in their diet or have suffered blood loss during dialysis. There is always some blood left over in the dialyzer (artificial kidney) once dialysis has ended. Over a long period of time, this can lead to anemia.

For those on dialysis, a renal dietitian might create a diet that excludes foods such as red meat and beans which are normally encouraged to help increase iron levels in the body. As a result, the body might develop anemia. A meal plan that includes other sources of iron that don't have a lot of protein can be created to improve iron levels in the body.

Symptoms of Anemia

Some of the symptoms of anemia can be confused with typical symptoms of chronic kidney disease. This is one of the reasons why informing your doctor of any new symptoms is so important. Symptoms of anemia can also differ depending on the severity. Anemia may occur without any symptoms at all and only be detected during a medical examination that includes blood work, especially if caught in the early stages of kidney failure.

Common symptoms of anemia can include:

- Fatigue
- Shortness of breath
- Pale skin
- Inability to think clearly
- Palpitations or rapid heartbeat
- Weakness
- Headache
- Ringing in ears (tinnitus)
- Loss of sexual desire
- Irritability
- Decreased appetite
- Cold hands and feet
- Depression

For many people, the first symptom of anemia is fatigue. They might start feeling tired and run down and notice that they have difficulty performing daily activities or work functions. Exercising or walking up and down stairs might leave them winded or exhausted. Over time, they may start feeling as though they just can't get enough sleep.

For others, along with the fatigue, there are general aches and pains and weakness. It might be hard to lift items that you didn't have trouble with in the past, to move things around, and to perform simple tasks. Some people lose their appetite or eat a few bites and then discover that they're not as hungry as they thought they were.

Many people find that they experience mental confusion or "brain fog." They have difficulty finding the right word that they want to use or can't remember what they were going to say or even what they did the day before. They feel restless, uncertain, and depressed. Their extremities feel cold and they have trouble getting warm when everyone else in the room doesn't seem to have a problem with the temperature. They lose interest in their favorite activities and look pale. They might experience hair loss or even weight loss.

These are all signs of anemia and anemia can affect every person a different way.

If anemia is left untreated, symptoms can include:

- A bluish tint to the whites of the eyes
- A sore mouth and tongue
- Brittle nails
- Restless leg syndrome (RLS) (tingling or crawling feeling in the legs)

- Changes in menstrual cycles
- Trouble achieving or maintaining an erection

Since the red blood cells transport oxygen to tissues and organs and enable them to utilize the energy they receive from food, any decreased oxygen levels may cause you to tire easily. The heart and brain can also suffer since they aren't getting the oxygen they need and this can make a person appear pale. Fatigue is one of the most common symptoms of anemia, simply for the reason that the body doesn't have the energy it needs in order to function properly.

There are some other symptoms of anemia, but these are considered rare. People with anemia sometimes develop pica, the medical condition that can cause an individual to crave substances that aren't food products, such as dirt, or to crave certain types of food such as those that are crunchy (raw vegetables or ice chips).

Anemia and left ventricular hypertrophy (LVH)

Left ventricular hypertrophy (LVH) is not a symptom of anemia, but can be a condition that is often associated with anemia and it's therefore important to mention it here. As the chamber that does all the pumping (the left ventricle), this muscle does a lot of work. When it becomes enlarged, as it can in response to anemia or other heart disease related conditions, it can cause a variety of symptoms.

A few of the factors that can cause LVH include:

- High blood pressure
- Anemia
- Heart problems

As the heart must work harder to pump, the chamber's walls grow thicker and this becomes a problem as they start losing their elasticity. It pumps harder because it does not have the oxygen it needs and cannot pump efficiently so it needs to pump more. This causes the heart to enlarge.

Symptoms of LVH can include:

- Shortness of breath
- Fatigue
- Chest pain

- Heart palpitations
- Dizziness
- Fainting

Over time, complications of left ventricular hypertrophy can develop if treatment is not sought. The overworked muscles can grow weaker and heart disease can develop. Heart disease is common in chronic kidney disease patients. Heart failure can also occur as the heart isn't able to receive a sufficient amount of oxygen. In addition, a heart attack can occur if there is an interruption of blood supply to the heart.

Lab tests

A complete blood count (CBC) is usually the first laboratory test that is performed when anemia is suspected. It is carried out on a sample of blood and includes a determination of an individual's hematocrit as well as the amount of hemoglobin in the blood. The CBC offers important information on the size, volume, and shape of the red blood cells.

Blood consists of plasma fluid, red blood cells, white blood cells, and additional kinds of cells. Your hematocrit tells the percentage of the blood that is made of red blood cells. Since blood cells can become diluted, those with a high volume of plasma (the liquid part of blood) can still be anemic. The National Kidney Foundation's Dialysis Outcome Quality

Initiative (K/DOQI) guideline recommends that the cause of anemia be figured out and treated in those whose hematocrit falls below 37% for post-menopausal women or 33% for women who menstruate. Anemia might also be diagnosed when hematocrit levels fall below:

- 36% for children 12 - 15 years
- 39% for adult men
- 36% for adult non-pregnant women
- 33% for adult pregnant women

Hemoglobin is the protein that contains iron and makes the blood red. It also carries the oxygen to the vital organs. For those with CKD, K/DOQI guidelines recommend an anemia work up carried out if hemoglobin falls below 12 g/dL (the "g/dL" stands for *grams per deciliter*) in post-menopausal women and men, 11 g/dL for pregnant women, 13 g/dL for men and 11 g/dL in women who menstruate. The lab tests for hemoglobin usually come back denoted as "Hgb."

Additional hemoglobin tests, such as mean corpuscular hemoglobin (MCH) and mean corpuscular hemoglobin concentration (MCHC) may also be taken during blood work. The mean corpuscular volume (MCV) measures the average size of red blood cells. It increases when red blood cells are bigger than normal (macrocytic) and it declines when the red blood cells are smaller than they should be (microcytic). The macrocytic cells can be signs of anemia that is brought on by a vitamin B12 deficiency. Microcytic cells are usually an indication of iron-deficiency anemia. Knowing this can help the doctor offer up the correct treatment.

The seriousness of anemia is categorized by the subsequent hemoglobin ranges:

- Mild anemia: between 9.5 - 13.0 g/dL
- Moderate anemia: between 8.0 - 9.5 g/dL
- Severe anemia: 8.0 g/dL

The doctor might also perform additional tests to determine if you have:

- A heart murmur
- Low blood pressure
- Rapid heart rate

Sometimes, if the doctor suspects internal bleeding, then additional tests could include an endoscopy. In this test, the patient is sedated and a camera is inserted into the stomach to look for internal bleeding and possible causes of blood loss.

When doing a blood test, the doctor will also be looking at the cause of anemia. As a result, additional blood tests can include:

- Blood levels of iron, vitamin B12, and folic acid
- Red blood count
- Reticulocyte count

People do have Hgb/Hct concentrations that might be standard for them, but be considered signs of anemia in comparison to the data for the general population. Conversely, some individuals have levels that may be insufficient for them despite the fact that they are considered standard. For that reason, other test results and even symptoms should be taken into consideration.

Knowing the reticulocyte count and iron parameters can be beneficial to determining the cause of anemia. A high reticulocyte count can imply that active hemolysis is present. In other words, the body just doesn't have enough healthy red blood cells. Active hemolysis means that the red blood cells live less than 100 days, instead of their standard 120. This can occur in acute renal failure thanks to the hemolytic uremic syndrome. If there is an irregular white blood cell count or abnormal platelet count then it might indicate a disturbance of bone marrow function.

Because iron is very important for hemoglobin synthesis, individuals should be assessed for the availability of iron in the body. This can be carried out by measuring the serum iron and the TIBC. These show the amount of iron that is on hand for hemoglobin synthesis; the serum ferritin shows the stored iron. If either of these are low then it might mean that the body needs an iron supplement to stimulate development of red blood cells.

There are two tests that can be used to determine if iron levels are low and both of these can be carried out during the Complete Blood Count.

The ferritin level shows the amount of iron that the body has stored. The ferritin score shouldn't be less than 100 micrograms per liter (mcg/L), nor greater than 800 mcg/L.

The TSAT indicates the transferrin saturation. This score shows how much iron the body has on hand in order to produce red blood cells. The score should be between 20-50%.

According to a report published by the Medical University of South Carolina in 1997, iron deficiency is present in as many as 37.5% of those who have anemia associated with chronic kidney disease. In most cases, iron deficiency is usually caused by blood loss, most commonly due to surgery. However, a stool test for blood is sometimes carried out to see if the patient has any gastrointestinal bleeding that could cause the iron deficiency.

For those individuals with chronic kidney disease who don't have an iron deficiency, it is necessary to look for other causes of anemia besides an erythropoietin deficiency.

Hypothyroidism can look like an EPO deficiency but is a very common cause of a normochromic (there's enough hemoglobin, just not enough red blood cells) and normocytic anemia (the red blood cells, hemoglobin, and hematocrit are all decreased).

Treating anemia

Treatment for anemia often depends on the type of anemia the patient is found to have. In some cases, simple iron supplements can be effective at managing anemia. Anemia in chronic kidney disease is often treated with an ESA, a laboratory-created protein that mimics the erythropoietin the body produces. This will boost red blood cell production. Brand names of EPO include EPOGEN and Procrit. Darbepoetin alfa is another ESA. It is long-acting and is usually only given once a week or once every other week. Vitamin B-12 and folic acid might also be given to the patient since these levels must be in a normal range in order for healthy red blood cell production to happen.

Historically, anemia has been treated with blood transfusions. This changed around 1990, though, when it started becoming more popular to treat anemia with different drug options. This was a welcomed relief to many since blood transfusions posed risks to patients, including allergic reactions and infections.

Erythropoiesis-stimulating agents (ESAs)

Those individuals who have anemia caused by low EPO are often prescribed erythropoiesis-stimulating agent (ESAs). Also referred to as "Epotein therapy," this is basically an injectable form of the EPO that healthy kidneys produce. It is typically injected under the skin at least twice a week and is generally administered in the doctor's office. Those on dialysis who are unable to take EPO shots may receive it at the same time they are getting their dialysis.

The ESA dose is generally adjusted every month until the Hgb is in the target range of 11-13 g/dL. Hgb levels are monitored at least once a month for patients taking these injections. The continued dosage will depend on the patient's needs and the doctor's discretion.

It is recommended by the U.S. Food and Drug Administration (FDA) that patients treated with ESA therapy should attain hemoglobin levels between 10 and 12 g/dL. There is a concern that raising the Hgb above 12 g/dL in those with CKD could increase the risk of stroke, heart attack, and even heart failure. If, during the blood work, it is discovered that the patient's Hgb level is above 12 g/dL, a lower dose is normally prescribed.

If you're taking an ESA, it's important to contact your doctor if you have any of the following symptoms:

- Pain in the legs
- Swollen legs
- Increased shortening of breath
- Escalating blood pressure

- Dizziness or fainting
- Fatigue or malaise
- Blood clots in the dialysis access ports

Although ESAs have been very successful at treating anemia in the past, there are some instances when they might not be as successful. An iron deficiency, for instance, can cause failure in the ESA therapy which is why iron levels should also be tested every month. Infection and inflammation can interact negatively with ESAs as well.

If the hemoglobin doesn't increase once the ESA treatment has begun, the doctor will usually check the iron levels again through more blood work. Although the level of erythropoietin in the body should be higher, the body still requires adequate iron to produce red blood cells. The iron is generally given in oral tablet form or can be administered through other means.

Almost all of the studies carried out on those who were on dialysis or predialysis and treated with Epoetin have demonstrated that with increased Hct, the individual has a better quality of life. Most individuals who undergo this therapy experience improved heart health, improved brain oxygen supply, more energy, more muscle strength, better cognitive function, better sleep, and a higher sexual function. The ability to exercise longer has been shown to increase when the Hct increases from 30% to 40%, according to a 1995 study published by the Kidney Center and Cardiology Section at the Shinraku-En Hospital in Niigata, Japan. For those with LVH, treating anemia with Epoetin resulted in partial regression of LVH in those on dialysis, according to a study published by the Canadian Erythropoietin Study Group at the Royal Victoria Hospital in Montreal.

In Epotein therapy, a 1998 Italian study noted an improved survival rate for those who had an Hct of more than 32%. In addition, a 1999 study published by the Nephrology Analytical Services through the Minneapolis Medical Research Foundation found that an Hct of 33% to 36% reduced the risk of death in comparison to those whose average Hct was 30% to 33%.

Iron Treatment

Iron supplements can be very helpful in treating anemia that is caused by low iron levels. However, only supplementing with iron will not be as beneficial if low iron is not the only cause of anemia.

A lot of patients with CKD require both ESA therapy and iron supplements. Supplemental iron is given in order to avoid iron deficiency and to help sustain sufficient iron stores so that the CKD patients can keep and hold Hgb 11 to 12 g/dL (Hct 33% to 36%) along with the ESA therapy.

If the patient's iron levels are very low, the ESAs won't be as helpful and the patient could continue to experience the symptoms associated with anemia. Iron tablets are sometimes the first course of action when a patient is diagnosed with anemia, until the cause of the anemia has been established. Even then, ESA therapy can be enhanced by iron supplements. Oral tablets usually contain at least 200 mg of elemental iron for adults.

Iron can also be administered through an injection. Sometimes, the doctor will test the patient with a small dose to ensure that they won't have a negative reaction. Negative reactions affect less than 1% of those who take them, so it's uncommon that the patient will experience anything adverse.

Since patients with CKD who are on dialysis can't always keep up with a sufficient iron level with oral tablets, they will usually receive iron supplements at the same time they are undergoing dialysis. Intravenous iron generally causes fewer stomach and intestinal pain.

Some patients experience headaches, muscle aches, and joint pain a couple of days after receiving the injection or IV treatment. These are generally treated with over the counter pain medications. For those who have trouble tolerating oral iron supplements, they may do better with smaller, more frequent doses. Some individuals also do better with iron tablets when they take them at bedtime, or when they start with a lower dose and then work their way up to something stronger.

Once the patient achieves a favorable Hgb/Hct and iron stores, a "maintenance" dose of iron can be given to help the patient maintain the levels they need. The TSAT and serum ferritin are monitored at least every three months to ensure that the iron stores are normal.

Ferrous and ferric are the two kinds of iron supplements. Most iron tablets contain ferrous iron since the body tends to absorb it better. It can come in three forms: ferrous gluconate, ferrous fumarate, and ferrous sulfate.

The tablet size is usually around 325 mg and the amount of elemental iron that the tablet contains is the amount of iron that is available for the body to absorb. Depending on the form of iron, a 325 mg iron supplement contains:

- Ferrous fumarate=108 mg of elemental iron

- Ferrous sulfate=65 mg of elemental iron

- Ferrous gluconate= 35 mg of elemental iron

Most of the time, a dosage of 60 - 200 mg of elemental iron per day is recommended, although this will also be dependent upon how bad the anemia. It's important to follow the prescription's directions and not take more iron than is prescribed in a daily dose.

There are some side effects of iron tablets. These can include:

- Black stools
- Nausea
- Vomiting
- Constipation
- Diarrhea

Both constipation and diarrhea are common side effects of taking iron supplements. Constipation is usually more predominant than diarrhea and your doctor might prescribe a gentle laxative. Other gastrointestinal problems such as vomiting and nausea may occur, too, especially with high doses of iron. For people who have stomach issues, ferrous gluconate is often a little gentler on the digestive system.

While black stools are common with iron supplements, it's important to make sure that you're not passing any blood in the stools. If the stools have a tarry look to them, or have bloody streaks, then it might be a sign of gastrointestinal bleeding and your doctor should be notified.

It is usually recommended that iron supplements be taken in between meals for better absorption, although ferrous sulfate tablets can be taken with food. It is also important to drink plenty of fluid, preferably water, when taking the tablets. Juices with vitamin C can be particularly helpful in absorption, but beware of orange juice with a potassium restriction. Some medications can actually hinder the absorption process so most pharmacists recommend waiting at least two hours after taking the supplement before taking any antacids or antibiotics.

Other tips for increasing your iron levels include:

- Don't take iron tablets at the same time that you take any phosphate binders.
- Take iron tablets between meals.
- If upset stomach occurs, take the iron tablets at bedtime.
- Don't take iron with alcohol, coffee, or milk.
- Only take the amount of iron that your doctor prescribes.
- Work with your renal dietitian to increase your intake of foods that are high in iron such as iron-fortified and iron-enriched cereals and enriched rice.

- Cook with an iron skillet. The iron from the skillet will be absorbed into some of the food, thus increasing your iron intake.

If low iron levels are the cause of the anemia, then the hemocrit should reach normal levels within two months of therapy. In most cases, to better manage the anemia, it is recommended that the iron therapy be continued for at least six months to help restore the bone marrow's iron stores.

Other supplements

For some individuals with CKD, supplements of vitamin B12 and folic acid may be necessary to treat and manage the anemia. Both of these levels must be normal in order for the body to produce red blood cells. Megalobastic anemia, for instance, is indicated by unusually large red blood cells and is caused by weakened absorption or a deficiency of vitamin B12 and folate. In this situation, the appropriate treatment typically involves a daily oral folic acid supplement. This should continue for a few months. It might also be recommended that the individual take vitamin B12 supplements or receive monthly injections.

Dietary changes

Working with your dietitian to make certain dietary changes might benefit some patients with anemia. Since the body absorbs iron best from protein sources, this can be a problem for those with CKD. Patients are generally advised to limit the amount of protein they consume. However, eating foods that are high in vitamin C can also help your body absorb iron better while other foods such as coffee and milk can actually hinder the absorption of iron. Your dietitian can help you create a meal plan that focuses on the foods that help your body absorb the iron you take in without eating anything that might be hard on your kidneys.

Iron rich foods

Iron can be discovered in foods that come from both plants and animals. The iron that is derived from animal sources is referred to as "heme" iron while the iron from plant sources is "nonheme" iron. Both sources are considered beneficial to the body. The body is able to absorb the iron that comes from animal sources better than it does from food sources, though. To create better absorption from plant foods, vitamin C can be helpful. The important thing for those with CKD is to choose foods that are right for their dietary plan while still getting the nutrients they need.

A healthy renal diet is meant to help the body maintain the proper balance of fluids, minerals, and nutrients. The diet is different for those who are on dialysis and those who aren't. Those who are predialysis are usually encouraged to limit protein while those who are undergoing dialysis usually require more protein in their diets.

Many protein-rich foods are also high in iron. Since low-protein diets are encouraged for those not on dialysis, those foods might not be suitable. Instead, your renal dietitian might recommend a moderate or low protein diet. Once you've started dialysis, however, foods that are higher in protein might be suggested. These foods, such as pork and eggs, can help replace any iron stores that might be depleted.

The following is a list of foods that are good sources of heme (animal based sources) iron:

- Chicken liver
- Oysters
- Clams
- Beef liver
- Lean ground beef
- Turkey leg
- Tuna
- Eggs
- Shrimp

These are good sources of nonheme (plant based sources) iron:

- Instant oatmeal
- Garlic
- Kidney beans
- Tofu
- Lentils
- Cranberries
- Molasses
- Whole wheat bread
- Peanut butter
- Brown rice
- Apricots
- Pineapple
- Raw broccoli

Combining both sources of iron foods with vitamin C at the same meal can increase the absorption of iron. For those on dialysis, vitamin C should be limited to 60 mg per day. There are kidney friendly vitamin C sources available. These include vitamin C enriched cranberry juice, strawberries, and tangerines.

Iron, Vitamin B12, & Folic Acid

The following foods are high in iron, vitamin B12, and folic acid. However, since patients with chronic kidney disease must also watch their potassium, the potassium amounts for each food are also listed beside each item. As you can see, some foods are good sources of iron, folic acid, and vitamin B12, they also contain a lot of potassium so should be limited if you are trying to limit or avoid potassium in your diet.

- Spinach ½ cup cooked=420 mg
- Sweet potatoes 1 with skin=450 mg
- Peas ½ cup=90 mg
- Broccoli ½ cup=230 mg
- Beet greens ½ cup 90 mg
- Kale 1 cup=300 mg
- Chard 480 mg
- Raisins ¼ cup=270 mg
- Iron-enriched cereals and grains (check the labels)
- Liver 1 oz=89 mg
- Artichokes 1 medium cooked=343 mg
- Strawberries 1 medium=18 mg
- Watermelon ½ cup=85 mg

- Dates 5=270 mg
- Tofu ½ cup=150 mg
- Beans (kidney, garbanzo, or white, canned) ½ cup=595 mg
- Tomato products (e.g., paste) ½ cup=275 mg
- Dried beans and peas ½ cup=300-475 mg
- Lentils ½ cup=365 mg
- Molasses 1 tbsp=195 mg
- Pineapple 1 cup=180 mg
- Brown rice 1 cup=85 mg
- Instant oatmeal 1 cup= 143 mg

Foods that are rich in vitamin B12 and their potassium levels include:

- Salmon 3 oz= 300 mg
- Tuna 3 oz=200 mg
- Crab 3 oz=225 mg
- Tofu ½ cup=150 mg
- Swiss cheese 1 slice=45 mg
- Eggs 1 hard boiled= 63 mg
- Oysters (6)= 215 mg
- 1 container of Greek, nonfat yogurt (8oz)= 240 mg
- Peach (1)= 285 mg
- Lobster 1 cup= 334 mg

Foods that are rich in Folic Acid and their potassium levels include:

- Egg yolk=19 mg
- Dried beans ½ cup=300-465 mg
- Lentils ½ cup=365 mg
- Almonds 1 oz =200 mg
- Sweet potato 1 baked with skin=450 mg
- Spinach ½ cup=420 mg
- Brussels sprouts ½ cup=250 mg
- Broccoli ½ cup=230 mg
- Banana (1)=425 mg
- Oranges (1)=240 mg
- Mustard greens 1 cup= 215 mg
- Asparagus 1 spear= 32 mg
- Strawberries (1)= 18 mg
- Carrots (1)=195 mg
- Squash 1 cup cubed= 406 mg
- Cabbage (1 leaf)= 39 mg

Being your own advocate

Most individuals with CKD are not able to avoid anemia completely. Still, you can work to manage it and, along with your healthcare team, do your best to ensure that it doesn't get worse. Sometimes this means that you must work as your own advocate, especially since you know your body better than anyone does.

Lab tests

It's important to know the results of your lab tests and understand what those results mean. You can ask for copies of them and then keep track of the results in your own file so that you know what your body is doing.

When you know and understand your lab test results you're an informed part of your own healthcare. It also allows you to talk to your healthcare team about any decisions in an educated manner and ask questions as they arise. When you know and understand your results, it permits you to follow any progress you're making over time, and this can be critical if you're taking any iron supplements or undergoing ESA therapy. Ask your doctor about what his or her goals are for your lab levels. Discuss the factors that can affect your results so you are able to make changes.

Ask questions

Never be afraid to ask questions when your healthcare is at stake. Some questions you might want to consider asking of your doctor include:

- What is my target level for each test?

- How long will I need to take each medication?

- How often will I be retested?

- How frequently will I need injections or IV treatment?

- Are there any known risks or side effects of this anemia treatment?

- Is there anything else I can be doing to manage my anemia?

- How can I bring my levels back to the target range?

- Why am I not being treated with ESAs or iron?

Asking questions allows you to know and understand what your doctor is trying to achieve and if you are reaching those goals. By you being proactive, your doctor will be more likely to keep you informed since you're showing interest. Of course, the biggest incentive to asking questions is that you'll learn the answers and will be able to act accordingly. These actions help you to get the best care as well.

Monitor your symptoms

When you are living with chronic kidney disease, it's important to keep track of your symptoms so that you know if anything is getting worse or improving. If you have new symptoms, they should be brought up to your medical team. When you have anemia, monitoring your symptoms is also important. This can let you know if your symptoms are linked to any lifestyle or dietary changes you're making or if they're associated with a certain medication. It will also let you know if the symptoms get better or worse as your lab results change.

Some people find that keeping a journal of their symptoms is helpful. You can keep track of new symptoms, when they occur, and if anything makes them worse or better. Taking this journal to your doctors' appointments can be beneficial since it might remind of you any questions or concerns you may have.

It can also help guide the decision making process of your doctor because they have more information to base the conclusion on.

Medication concerns

As a patient with CKD, you might have several different medications that you are taking. Because keeping track of all of them might be difficult, and then when you add your anemia medication on top of them it might become even more confusing, listing them out is very helpful.

By keeping track of medications, you'll be informed and understand what you're taking and why. A journal with a schedule might be helpful when it comes to taking your medications at the right time and in the proper way (For instance, iron supplements at bedtime). A benefit of this is that you might avoid some of the side effects associated with certain medications and the medications themselves might even be more effective since you're taking them correctly. It also can help caregivers when they need to administer medications. Keeping the information in a spiral notebook with dates and times taken can be helpful to remembering what you have taken – or provide a great deal of assistance to your caretaker.

Conclusion

For those individuals with chronic kidney disease, managing anemia is critical when it comes to improving their quality of life and overall health. Anemia management in those with kidney disease can help prevent or improve such symptoms as fatigue and mental cognition and even decrease the risk of being hospitalized.

It's important to talk to the members of your health care team about proper anemia lab tests and management of the condition. Those who have both CKD and anemia have a higher risk for stroke and heart problems and even an increased risk of death. If you also have diabetes, then the risk of these are even greater.

Naturally, your health care team is responsible for providing you with the best care management possible. Still, it's up to the individual patient to be their own advocate where their health is concerned. This means following through with treatments, informing your healthcare provider of any new symptoms or issues, taking prescribed medications in the correct manner, and sticking to the diet that the renal dietitian has prescribed.

It's always important to ask any questions you have of your healthcare provider and to raise concerns as they arise. In addition, it's important to understand why you're being prescribed something and to know what's going on inside your body. If something doesn't feel right, then listen to your body, then talk to your healthcare team, and make sure that you and your healthcare provider are on the same page.

Other Titles By Mathea Ford:

Mathea Ford, Author Page (all books):

http://www.amazon.com/Mathea-Ford/e/B008E1E7IS/

The Kidney Friendly Diet Cookbook

http://www.amazon.com/Kidney-Friendly-Diet-Cookbook-PreDialysis-ebook/dp/B00BC7BGPI/

Create Your Own Kidney Diet Plan

http://www.amazon.com/Create-Your-Kidney-Diet-Plan-ebook/dp/B009PSN3R0/

Living with Chronic Kidney Disease - Pre-Dialysis

http://www.amazon.com/Living-Chronic-Kidney-Disease-Pre-Dialysis-ebook/dp/B008D8RSAQ/

Eating a Pre-Dialysis Kidney Diet - Calories, Carbohydrates, Fat & Protein, Secrets To Avoid Dialysis

http://www.amazon.com/Eating-Pre-Dialysis-Kidney-Diet-Carbohydrates-ebook/dp/B00DU2JCHM/

Eating a Pre-Dialysis Kidney Diet - Sodium, Potassium, Phosphorus and Fluids, A Kidney Disease Solution

http://www.amazon.com/Eating-Pre-Dialysis-Kidney-Diet-Phosphorus-ebook/dp/B00E2U8VMS/

Eating Out On a Kidney Diet: Pre-dialysis and Diabetes: Ways To Enjoy Your Favorite Foods

http://www.amazon.com/Eating-Out-Kidney-Diet-Pre-dialysis/dp/0615928781/

Kidney Disease: Common Labs and Medical Terminology: The Patient's Perspective

http://www.amazon.com/Kidney-Disease-Terminology-Perspective-Pre-Dialysis/dp/0615931804/

Dialysis: Treatment Options for the Progression to End Stage Renal Disease

http://www.amazon.com/Dialysis-Treatment-Options-Progression-Disease/dp/0615932258/

Mindful Eating For A Pre-Dialysis Kidney Diet: Healthy Attitudes Toward Food and Life

http://www.amazon.com/Mindful-Eating-Pre-Dialysis-Kidney-Diet/dp/0615933475/

The Emotional Challenges Of Coping with Chronic Kidney Disease

http://www.amazon.com/Emotional-Challenges-Chronic-Disease-Dialysis-ebook/dp/B00H6SYQG8/

Heart Healthy Living with Kidney Disease: Lowering Blood Pressure http://www.amazon.com/Heart-Healthy-Living-Kidney-Disease/dp/0615936059/

Exercising with Chronic Kidney Disease: Solutions To An Active Lifestyle

http://www.amazon.com/Exercising-Chronic-Kidney-Disease-Solutions/dp/0615936342/

Sexuality and Chronic Kidney Disease For Men and Women: A Path To Better Understanding

http://www.amazon.com/Sexuality-Chronic-Kidney-Disease-Women/dp/0615960197/

Sign up for our email list to learn of new titles right away!

http://www.renaldiethq.com/go/email/

www.ingramcontent.com/pod-product-compliance
Lightning Source LLC
Chambersburg PA
CBHW070947210326
41520CB00021B/7100